DEPRESSION

Learn About Teen Depression Signs and Treatment

I0486166

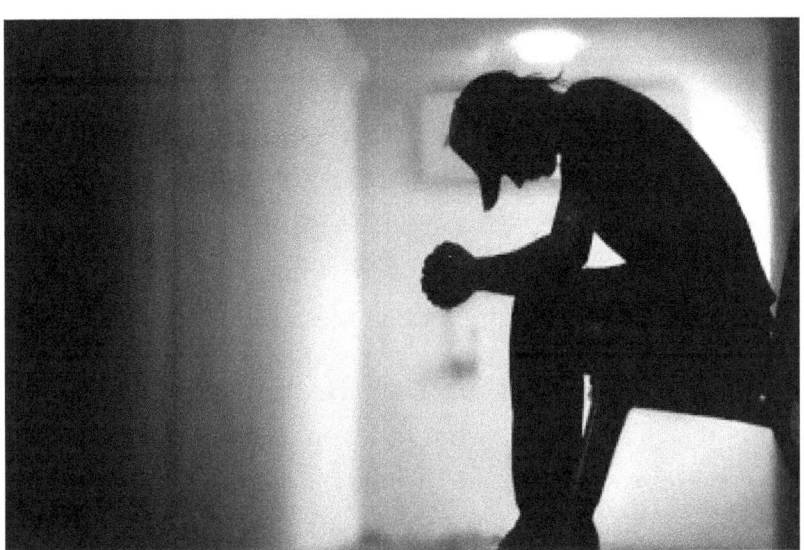

By Patricia A Carlisle

Introduction

I want to thank you and congratulate you for choosing the book, "*DEPRESSION: Learn About Teen Depression Signs and Treatment*".

This book contains proven steps and strategies on how to recognize the signs of depression in teens, and what treatment will help them to combat their symptoms.

Depression can cause a person to function at a low level, especially when the person is being affected by psychological depression which can lead to being sad, inactive, having difficulty in thinking, and not being able to concentrate; they show a significant increase or decrease in appetite, and spend a lot of time sleeping, feeling of hopelessness, and sometimes suicidal tendencies are all associated with depression.

We are going to focus on Teen Depression, the signs and treatment. Therefore, what is teen depression? When a teenager is growing up, and when the younger person begins to encounter situations and circumstances that the individual has never experienced before, beginning from the basic unit of life (i.e. the family and to the larger contemporary society) . The teenager may not be experienced on how to handle the problem which often can lead to depression, and the above mentioned symptoms of depression begins to develop, and take its toll on the them.

Thanks again for choosing this book, I hope you enjoy it!

© Copyright 2017 by Holistic Measures, LLC- All rights reserved.

This document is geared towards providing exact and reliable information in regards to the topic and issue covered. The publication is sold with the idea that the publisher is not required to render accounting, officially permitted, or otherwise, qualified services. If advice is necessary, legal or professional, a practiced individual in the profession should be ordered.

- From a Declaration of Principles which was accepted and approved equally by a Committee of the American Bar Association and a Committee of Publishers and Associations.

In no way is it legal to reproduce, duplicate, or transmit any part of this document in either electronic means or in printed format. Recording of this publication is strictly prohibited and any storage of this document is not allowed unless with written permission from the publisher. All rights reserved.

The information provided herein is stated to be truthful and consistent, in that any liability, in terms of inattention or otherwise, by any usage or abuse of any policies, processes, or directions contained within is the solitary and utter responsibility of the recipient reader. Under no circumstances will any legal responsibility or blame be held against the publisher for any reparation, damages, or monetary loss due to the information herein, either directly or indirectly.

Respective authors own all copyrights not held by the publisher.

The information herein is offered for informational purposes solely, and is universal as so. The presentation of the information is without contract or any type of guarantee assurance.

The trademarks that are used are without any consent, and the publication of the trademark is without permission or backing by the trademark owner. All trademarks and brands within this book are for clarifying purposes only and are the owned by the owners themselves, not affiliated with this document.

ABOUT THE AUTHOR

Patricia A. Carlisle, MSW, CBT

Patricia Carlisle- a Master Social Worker and Cognitive Behavioral Therapist (CBT) gives out an expression of how important it is for an individual to take into consideration the concept of self-assessment to know what human, technical and conceptual skills they posses to perform or to achieve what they desire, or to deal with everyday life. However, every particular group of people has their own unique set of ideas, traditions and events including the frame of mind according to which people perform but there are many who faces problems and fail to maintain a healthy mind set affecting their behaviors and performance to those around them.

People like Patricia Carlisle are among those who have felt this urge of serving people and helping them out of their mental crisis towards a healthy life. She has experienced some close encounters in her personal life regarding mental health issues in her family and friends that has encouraged her to pursue this as her career.

Currently Patricia Carlisle is serving as a Certified On-Line Cognitive Behavioral Therapist with an extensive 15years of experience using Cognitive-Behavior Therapy Techniques. She envisions a world where everyone gets mental health treatment with no mental health stigma and to make it real she has already set up her own Holistic Measure Online Comprehensive Behavioral Healthcare Company after retiring from The Nord Center in The Partial Hospitalization Program (PHP) Dept for 5 years and Murtis H. Taylor Mental Health Center as a mental health counselor, psychological support technician and case manager for 10 years to emulsify her skills more professionally.

Along with this, she has wrote down her passion as a clinician in 25 or more short books to help individuals and families get their life back, freeing them of the restraints of negative thinking, anxiety and depression by using different approaches. She is highly appreciated among her clients for her flexibility and professionalism of dealing with them graciously. To reach her, make use of her direct website address: http://therapist2013.wix.com/e-therapy . As she is ready to inspire hope and contribute to health and well-being by providing the best online health care through comprehensive practice, education and research.

TABLE OF CONTENT

Chapter 1

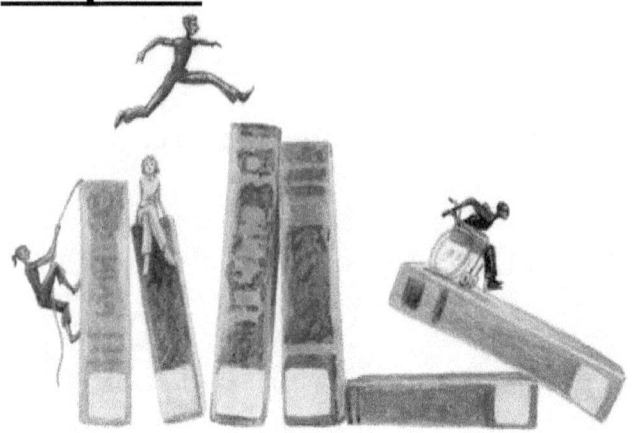

CHALLENGES FOR TEENS

Growing up as a teenager is very challenging, and sometimes the circumstances faced by a teenager if not properly managed can be very dangerous. For instance, when an adolescent is growing up and began to move into the larger society, from the schools or colleges that he or she attends, there are chances that he can be lured and introduced to dangerous social vices like smoking, alcoholism, gangs just to mention a few. Most teens sometimes get bullied in schools and that can lead to psychological depression, the fear of the threat by these bullies scares them so much that they find it difficult to talk about the horrible experiences to their parents.

Some parents may not be able to spend quality time with their children to find out what difficulties they are facing as they are growing up due to the parents career, or busy work schedule. Psychologically, depression as experienced by a teenager can linger for a very long time, and when this happens, the horrible experiences can transmit into adulthood, and may become very difficult to stop the problem when the teenager is gradually advancing in age.

Chapter 2

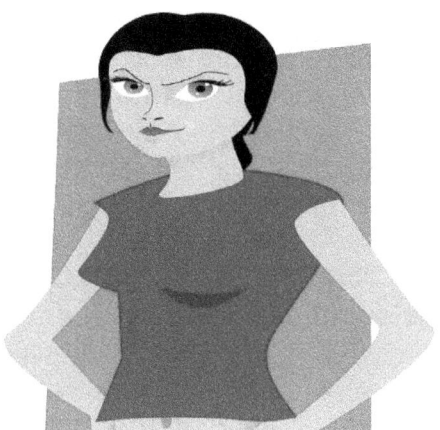

WHEN TEENS GET DEPRESSED

So how and why do teens get depressed? When it is noticeable that a teenager easily gets irritated, or feels unhappy then it is likely that the youngster is experiencing what is referred to as teen depression. Teens are very sensitive, and their emotion sometimes swings like the pendulum fixed in a specific position. There has been many feasibility studies on teens, it was discovered that they all possess similar tendencies when it comes to emotional disposition. It is a universal phenomenon that one out of at least ten teenagers is undergoing some form of depression.

However, depression can be taken care of, but that does not imply that there are no consequences, or adverse effects of making efforts to treat teen depression. Therefore, when you observe that a teenager is not happy, and the expression on his or her face and attitude is not right, or there are certain characteristics, and other symptoms being displayed by the teenager that continues for a minimum period of two weeks, then you need to get involved, and determine what issues the teen is going through. You may not necessarily have to take the matter into your own hands in finding out the problem. But you can talk to a health professional who will be able to offer adequate solution. Sometimes parents go for therapist who are skilled and have knowledge about problems associated with teens.

If you are wondering why teenagers get depressed, then it might surprise you to know that there are a thousand and one reasons why the situation of the teenagers can lead to depression. Some of the reasons are some teenagers are capable of building negative feelings of being worthless, and develop inferiority complex over their peer groups. Also, educational performances, sexual orientation, social status among their colleagues or their parents, lifestyle and family background, and many more are some of the factors that can affect how a teenager is feeling at a particular point in time. Teenage stress can also come from some environmental factors commonly referred to as environmental stress or depression. If a teen is in a good environment, and everything that he or she needs is provided, and yet the teenager is still not happy, or is feeling sad all the time, and continue to isolate themselves, then this is a very clear sign of teenage depression.

Chapter 3

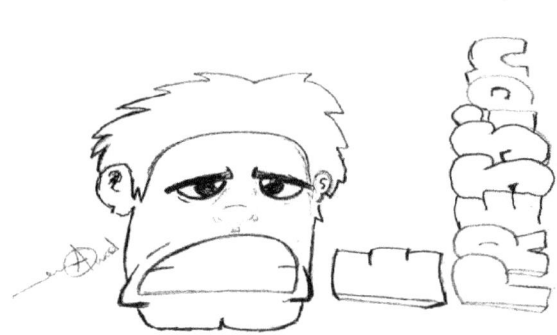

SIGNS OF TEEN DEPRESSION

Teenagers should be happy all the time; they do not have the weight of a huge task or responsibilities, especially when they have parents or guardian. The major duty they owe themselves is to take advantage of the educational provisions given to them by their parents or the government. However, when it is obvious and noticeable that there is a change in the thinking and behavior of a child, then like I stated earlier, you can begin to suspect depression. You will notice they do not have much motivation, and many times they tend to withdraw themselves from normal interactions, going to their room, and closing their doors after school hours, and remaining indoors for many hours.

ENGAGING IN EXCESSIVE SLEEPING

It is the characteristics of many teens who are depressed to sleep for several hours, sometimes they tend to have a change in their eating habits, some have the tendencies of not eat much food, and are not interested, or lack the appetite to eat. While in some teens the resultant effect of depression can be a sharp change in eating habit, they can eat a lot without watching their weight gain, and the risk of obesity that can become a problem at the end of the day.

CRIMINAL ACTIVITIES

Depression in teenagers can lead to anti-societal habits, or lead them to criminal activities. Some unhealthy activities common among teenagers with depression is shoplifting. Teenage shoplifting is on the rise every year, and this continue to constitute a major problem in cities around the world. When you notice a teenager is engaging in these unhealthy habits or activities, try to talk to them to find out if depression can be found.

PHYSICAL PAIN

When the teenager constantly complains of pains and having headaches, tiredness, and stomach aches, and after medical examination the doctor cannot find anything wrong, but yet he or she still feels these symptoms, then it could be a clear case of teenager depression. Often times, when a youngster is having difficulty in concentrating in his academic studies, it tends to affect the overall performances of the teenager. When they experience the lack of concentration it's very necessary for parents, teachers or guardian to take drastic steps to try to solve the problem, because this stage in the life of a teenager is very critical. The child's education should not be sacrifice on the "altar of depression". Hence, the matter should not be handled with "kid's glove". Therefore, when a child is having a hard time concentrating on his or her studies, then it is possible they could be suffering from teenage depression. Also, when a teenager is having difficulty in making decisions, especially when the teenager is always making the wrong decision, or is not capable of making an independent decision free from influence of the opinion of others, then there is a problem.

EXCESSIVE FEELINGS OF GUILT

Teenage depression comes in diverse dimensions, while looking at the face of a teenager an adult can read between the lines. The excessive feeling of guilt is inappropriate for a normal teenager. But when it is obvious, and noticeable that a teen is constantly feeling guilty and readily apologizes for what he or she feels guilty about unnecessarily, the possibilities of teenage depression is developing in such a teenager. A teenager may excessively feel guilty if he or she feels they are disappointing their parents, an unhealthy behavior can develop between the child and the parents, this can lead to the teen becoming a runaway; this is a situation where the teenager wonders away from home or family. The street is dangerous for a teenager, the youngster can be exposed to dangerous gangs that engage in criminal activities, or even the child may become a victim of crime.

STRANGE BEHAVIOR

When a teenager develops strange behavior such as becoming forgetful of simple responsibilities, obligations or task, or assignment given to him or her, this could be the start of teen depression, and if the young person is in the habit of coming late to classes, and becoming truant; avoiding or skipping school, and shows little or no interest in fostering his or her educational pursuit, the danger of teenage depression has already began to take its roots on the teenager. Lacking the appetite for food, or drastic loss of weight which obviously makes the teenager look thin, and you begin to wonder whether the child is deliberately avoiding food, or that he or she has a diet problem, your assumptions can be wrong when the main reason for this is the child is suffering from teenage depression.

MEMORY LOSS

Many teenagers also experience memory loss when they are depressed. It is not that they do not read, even if they become "bookworms" when the problem of depression sets in, no matter the length of time spent in reading, the lack of concentration will never allow them to have any meaningful impact as a result of depression. This can also cause low performance in their academic activities. When the teenager begin to have nightmares, when he or she constantly dreams of death or dying, when this occurs every night and they begins to have the feeling of insecurity ,and always from the belief that someone is after their life (paranoid), definitely there is a psychological imbalance, and can cause teenage depression.

Chapter 4

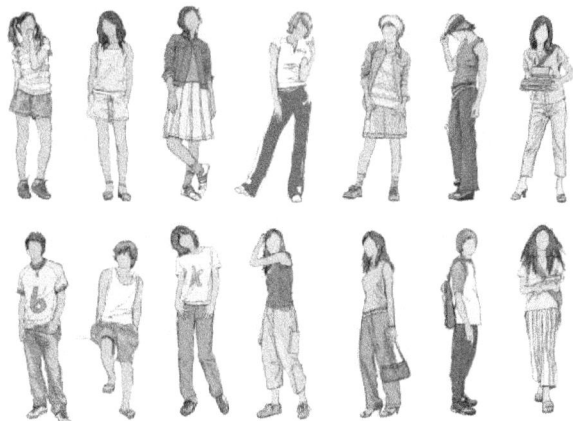

THE REBELIOUS TEENAGER

We have rebellious teenagers in every society, you want to know more? Then visit WELFARE HOMES FOR CHILDREN, and you will be surprise to see the number of teenagers who are left there. These children continue to increase in numbers, their parents are unable to cope with their stubborn and rebellious attitudes, and the only option some parents feel they have is sending these kids to government owned CHILD WELFARE. In some underdeveloped countries, there are no adequate facilities to aid in correction of the abnormal behaviors of some of these teens.

They end up being hard criminals, and the so called WELFARE HOMES unfortunately becomes a breeding ground for future hard criminals. These kids often developed hatred for their parents for abandoning them at the welfare homes without care, and when they come out they can be very dangerous, but that is for the underdeveloped countries. On the other hand, for developed nations they may have good facilities, and the skilled man power to take care of these groups of teenagers who are going through depression.

The feeling of hopelessness, sadness and anxiety is a clear indication that a teenager is undergoing depression, and the parents have to do everything within their powers to make sure they are helping more to find out if teenage depression is affecting the child. If you witness a sudden drop in a teenager's grades, and the youngster is also engaged in alcoholism, drugs, and develops promiscuous sexual habits, and having bad influential friends, not of parental approval, and withdraws from good friends, then the teenager could be undergoing depression.

Teenage Depression should be taken seriously, because when depression takes place, the next thing that follows is psychological and health complications, then the ultimate thing that crowns their mind is the options of suicide. Now it might interest you to know that it is universally confirmed that all individuals who commit suicide are those who are DEPRESSED, their depression has hit the limits, and the act is committed at the high point. I'm sure that is not what any parents want for their kids. There are so many other signs of teenage depressions and causes so be aware.

Chapter 5

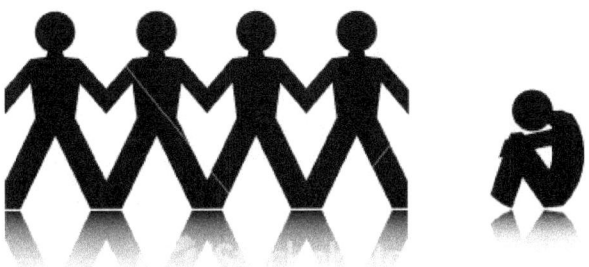

HOW TO DEAL WITH TEEN DEPRESSION

Before we can treat teenage depression, there are some elements of facts we need to know. If you do not have the time as a parent, you can find the services of experts who have the skills to handle such cases.

UNDERSTANDING

We need to understand an adult mind is very different from a teenager's mind. The way the adult perceives or conceives situations is not the same as a teen will receive similar information most of the time. So we need a lot of patients, diligence, and care to be able to treat a teenager who is depressed. Firstly, we need to encourage the depressed teenager to open up, and feel free to discuss the problem. You need to make some efforts by coming down to the teen's level of understanding and insight. You can start by becoming his or her friend; make the teen feel that you can be trusted. When a teenager is depressed, and if not, try to get to the root of the problem to salvage the situation whether it is depression or not. In that way, you would stop impending depression before it gets started. Thus, you will have to do in a loving, and not in a judgmental approach, encouraging the child to share the problem with you and let them know that you are concerned with the changes in his or her behavior.

TRUST

Sometimes, teens may not be comfortable in sharing their problems, because they are not sure of what reaction they may get from you, or they could be shy, afraid, or been threatened by a third party not to disclose any information or else they will get hurt. So that is the reasons you need to make the child be able to trust you. The teen may not realize that he is depressed, but your right about the teen's situation, so offer to let the child know your there for him or her unconditionally. You don't need to ask too many questions, but be supportive because teenagers find it difficult to cope with being clouded with questions, and they often feel insecure by excessive questions.

EXPRESS YOUR CONCERNS

Be gentle while expressing concern about the teen; do not intrude on the child's comfort zone while the teen is trying to cooperate with you. If the teen shuts you out, do not give up, try to buy yourself some time, and make him or her feel relaxed when both of you are interacting. Try to show your concern, and don't try to control his or her words, or responses always express the willingness to listen to whatever he or she has to say. Avoid the rush to criticize, or passing judgment once the teenager begins to communicate. Do not give any standing order or advice that may jeopardize your conversation with the youngster because that could ruin the communication between you and the teen. Accept the child deposition even if you feel it is irresponsible, or that his irrational behavior is unacceptable. But acknowledge his feelings, and your willingness to help out no matter what the situation is. Make the child see the reasons you are taking him seriously.

TAKE ACTION

Depression can be so damaging, when you notice the signs do not think that it will go away naturally. You need to take drastic action immediately, by seeking professional advice, or go through the necessary steps as listed above. If you are relying on a professional, make the necessary appointments for the child with a therapist for depression screening. Be ready to share depressive signs exhibited by your child to the therapist; that should include the length of time the child has been having such behavioral traits and the impact, or extent it has affected the child whether it was on daily basis, weekly, monthly etc. the pattern of behavioral changes.

If it is a situation where depression is something that has to do with heredity, then a physician is suitable for this kind of depression. A medical examination is needed such as blood sample, medical causes, and parental history. This is the responsibilities of the physician to determine. A medical health professional who has advance skills and quality background in treating teenagers in this regard is the best person for the teen's best care.

Chapter 6

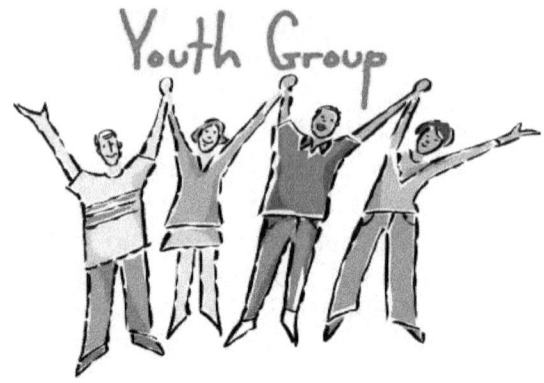

TREATMENT AND CARE

Although there is no single adequate care in treating teenage depression, it sometimes requires all hands to be on deck. The parents, the child, the specialist combining efforts will always be to the best interest of the child. And as we all know these steps are taken, and yet the child is still not connecting, there are other options that can be recommended by professionals in the field of managing adolescents, reach out and seek their advices to make sure you have explored all available resources for the best interest of the child. Treating teenage depression cannot be relied upon by medication alone. You need to explore other scientific and social means available. One on one talk, family therapy, and environmental changes can also be deplored.

Some people recommend antidepressant usage. This is still being introduced only to the adults; it has not been certified to be administered on children due to safety concerns because of the unknown measures to be taken. The teenage brain is very sensitive. You can support a teenager with some activities that will assist in treating depression such as:

o Giving them the environment to participate in physical or sporting activities allowing them to interact with other children. If you allow them to be in isolation at home all the time, you are not helping matters. So allow them a healthy environment that will help them to develop adequately.

o Allow them to have social activities, such as birthday parties, visit good friends, and going to game centers.

o And above all, engage them in useful academic activities that will improve their minds.

o Encourage them to read novels. You should also make time to get involve, and monitor the progress of your child.

o Try to learn more about teenage depression, read about it, and visit experts and therapist with your child to learn causes associated with teenage depression.

Conclusion

Thank you again for choosing this book!

I hope this book was able to help you to identify and learn about teen depression, signs and treatment.

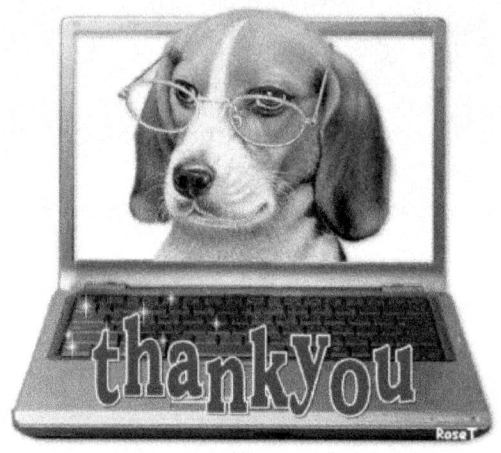

Finally, if you enjoyed this book, would you be kind enough to leave a review for this book on Amazon? It'd be greatly appreciated!

Thank you and good luck!

Preview Of 'HOW TO LIVE WITH PEOPLE AFFECTED WITH MENTAL ILLNESS'

Chapter 1: INTRODUCTION

Stigma associated with mental illness and psychiatric treatment, and the discrimination towards people with mental illnesses that frequently results from this, are the main obstacles preventing early and successful treatment. To reduce such stigma and discrimination towards mentally ill people and especially those with schizophrenia, the World Psychiatric Association's (WPA) anti stigma programmed 'Open the Doors' is currently being implemented in more than 20 countries. The programmed has been undertaken in seven project centers in Germany. Public information programs and education measures aimed at selected target groups are intended to improve the public's knowledge regarding symptomatolgy, causes and treatment options for

schizophrenia.

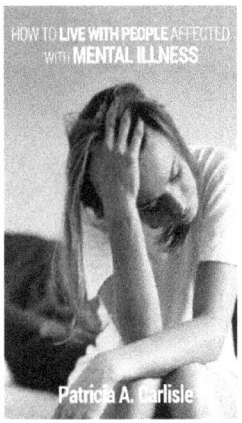

How to live with people affected with mental illness.

Check Out My Other Books

Below you'll find some of my other popular books that are popular on Amazon and Kindle as well. Alternatively, you can visit my author page on Amazon to see other work done by me. (https://amazon.com/author/patriciacarlisle)

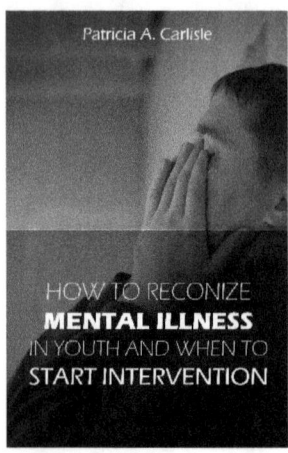

How to Recognize Mental Illness in Youth and When to Start Intervention.

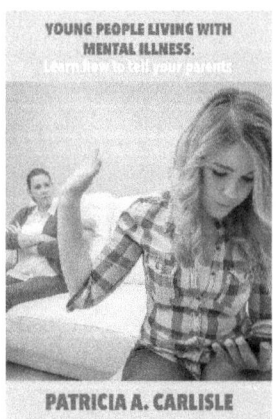

YOUNG PEOPLE LIVING WITH MENTAL ILLNESS: Learn How To Tell Your Parents.

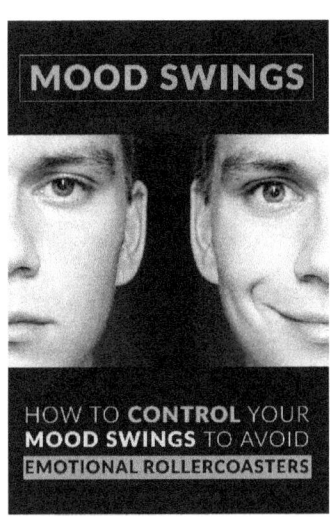

Mood Swings: How to control your mood swings to avoid emotional rollercoster's.

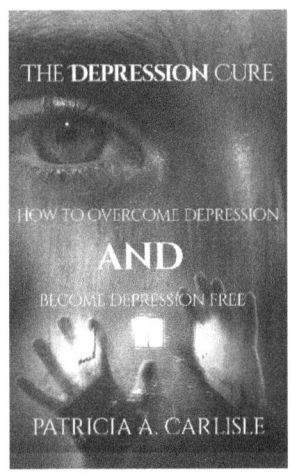

THE DEPRESSION CURE: How to overcome depression and become depression free.

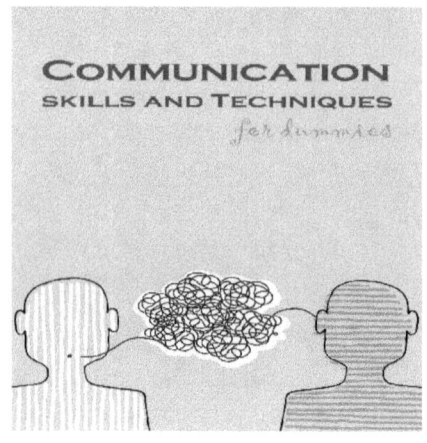

COMMUNICATION SKILLS AND TECHNIQUES FOR DUMMIES.

BONUS: SUBSCRIBE TO THE FREE BOOK

Beginners Guide to Yoga & Meditation

"Stressed out? Do You Feel Like The World Is Crashing Down Around You? Want To Take A Vacation That Will Relax Your Mind, Body And Spirit? Well this Easy To Read Step By Step

E-Book Makes It All Possible!"

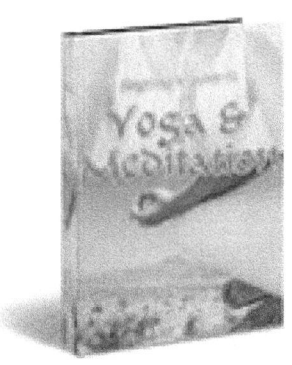

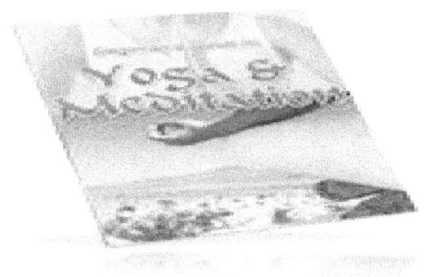

Instructions on how to join our mailing list, and receive a free copy of "Yoga and Meditation" can be found in any of my Kindle eBooks.

NOTES

NOTES

NOTES

NOTES

NOTES

NOTES

NOTES

NOTES

www.ingramcontent.com/pod-product-compliance
Lightning Source LLC
Chambersburg PA
CBHW070748180526
45168CB00004B/1565